**Copyright © 2019**
**Andrea Thompson**

**andreathompson.org • howibeatcancer.net**

Cover photos provided by: Heather Armstrong
heatherarmstrongphotography.com

Makeup provided by: Rachel McKnew

## A Word of Thanks

My life and the redemptive message behind it wouldn't be possible without these incredible people:

My husband, Joe
My kids
Dr. Raymond Hilu
Dr. Ken Adams
Robin Cook
Dr. Inge Wetzel
Dr. Amanda Campbell
Dr. Charles Majors
Tammy Roach
Jon Essen
My friends and family that supported me, prayed for me and stuck by me during all that I've been through.

And really, most of all, Jesus. He's always everything I need, when I need it.

# Table of Contents

## Foreword

Health is an ever-changing journey, one that people have been on since the beginning of time. God could have created our bodies to be self-sufficient vessels, never needing to rely on anything other than Him to survive. He chose, instead, to give us the ability to use food to nourish ourselves. He gave us free will.

In 2018, I was diagnosed with breast cancer. It was a shock to say the least. I had written a book on health and took good care of myself through diet and exercise. Apparently, there were underlining causes, but I wouldn't learn that until later on in my journey back to health. At this time in my life, I was friends with Andrea, but very soon she would become more than a friend. She would become my health coach, helping to walk me through this season of my life.

She was a Godsend to me. I had no grid for what I was about to go through. Andrea was there not only with encouragement, but also with extensive knowledge. She had gone through her own cancer journey and knew the what, when, where and how of what I would be going through. After I had a complete double mastectomy, I decided to use holistic healing to continue my process. Andrea knew right where to go. She connected me with Dr. Hilu in Spain, and I immediately started on a healing protocol with him. Eventually, Andrea and I would go to Spain together for holistic treatments.

Throughout this whole journey, Andrea was there. At every point, I leaned on her knowledge and experience. This was particularly true when it came to my emotional health. We are a triune being—body, soul and spirit— and these three must work beautifully together in order for us to walk in complete health. Going through a diagnosis like this, however, can feel like riding an emotional roller coaster. Andrea lent me her strength. There were days that were good, emotionally, where I felt strong and sure. And then there were days when the lies would come. It was so good to have Andrea there, telling me that she knew exactly what I was going through. It meant so much to connect and realize I would get through this. Right now, I am on the other side—cancer free, maintaining a healthy protocol to keep it that way.

The journey to our health is not for the weak at heart, and it must be a decision that each person makes for themselves. I learned that, in order to make real and lasting changes, I needed to make sacrifices that come with a price. I had to learn to say "No" to my flesh's cravings in order to serve a greater "Yes" towards honoring God with my body.

Our bodies are a gift that God has given each of us. The Bible goes as far as calling our bodies the temple of the Holy Spirit. What an honor to be entrusted with His temple.

I love the revelation that my friend, Andrea, has been given. Her journey has been nothing short of a challenge from which she has emerged victorious. Pursuing health and finding good, holistic approaches can get overwhelming. I think that one of the main questions I get from people is, "Where do I start? There's so much information out there today."

From my own experience, I highly recommend both my friend and my health coach, Andrea Thompson. If you are looking for wisdom in your own health journey, I believe that Andrea's insight and knowledge are going to

be the lighthouse that leads people back to their original
design in health.

To your health,

Beni Johnson
Bethel Church, Redding, CA
Author of *Healthy & Free* and *The Power of Communion*

## A Disclaimer and an Encouragement

This book offers health, fitness and nutritional information and is designed for educational purposes only. You should not rely on this information as a substitute for, nor does it replace, professional medical advice, diagnosis or treatment. If you have any concerns or questions about your health, you should always consult with a physician or other healthcare professional. Do not disregard, avoid or delay obtaining medical or health related advice from your health care professional because of something you may have read within this book. The use of any information provided within this book is solely at your own risk.

Developments in medical research may impact the health, fitness and nutritional advice that appears here. No assurance can be given that the advice contained in this book will always include the most recent findings or developments with respect to the particular material.

That being said, the information found within this book radically changed my life, and ultimately, my health.

In short, it saved my life.

As you read, I want you to be encouraged by my journey and consider the principles and protocols I share.

You should consult your physician or other healthcare professional before applying these principles and protocols to determine if they are right for your needs.

Believing for better health in your life,

Andrea Thompson

## My Cancer Wake-Up Call

Cancer.

It's an ugly word.

The word in itself tends to bring an onslaught of emotions ranging from anger, pain, and most of all, fear. Our society has learned to think of cancer as a death sentence rather than a diagnosis.

I can't say I blame them. The most common methods of treatment are chemotherapy and radiation and even those have a success rate of only 2-10%.

When the treatments alone significantly decrease your quality of life, who wants to even take those chances? The reality is that many people do. We've been conditioned to believe that those methods are our only chance to survival.

Allow me to first say that I have the utmost respect for doctors and their medical care. Many doctors go into the profession because of their desire to help people and see them live to their fullest potential.

However, modern medicine does not always allow them to do just that.

On August 1, 2012 I was at the Phoenix airport waiting to board a flight to California. It was then that I received a phone call at 8:30am that many of us pray we never receive.

My doctor of over 20 years called to tell me that I had cervical cancer. My vision blurred and my mind raced as the words he spoke began to become jumbled in my disbelief. The airport that was just a few minutes ago busy and loud seemed to have gone completely silent and motionless. I kept trying to think of ways to rewind time and take the words back that he said, but I couldn't.

I couldn't have cancer. I had already had to overcome so much in my life. To give you perspective, I was molested by a family member as a child, gang raped as a teenager, abandoned by my father in my late teens, gained and lost 100 pounds, battled an eating disorder, forced into the sex industry as a stripper, and survived a horrific divorce all by the age of 35.

As you could see, my life had been anything but easy. Couldn't life give me this free pass considering I had children to raise and had only been married to my now husband for three years? I had so much life ahead of me!

Cancer is no respecter of persons. It doesn't only happen to "other" people. It could happen to anyone. Even myself, someone who prided myself on being healthy and a Taekwondo instructor at the time, could get it.

I sat in my doctor's office while he went into detail about my diagnosis and that's when he broke the news to me.

"Andrea," he said with sadness in his eyes. "If you don't follow traditional protocol, including chemotherapy and radiation, at best you have a year to live."

The Bible makes it clear that we do not know the time or the hour when any of us shall pass, but hearing the words "a year to live" shook me to my core.

I drove home with thoughts running through my mind. How was my husband going to respond to the fact that his wife had cancer? What would my children do without their mother? How would I be able to fulfill everything that my heart desired to accomplish? How was this fair?

The fact that I even had cancer hadn't had time to settle with me yet.

> *I knew that I had a decision to make. I decided that cancer doesn't have to be a death sentence.*

I could either listen to my doctor's orders and undergo the harsh treatment of chemotherapy and radiation, or I could fight it naturally and according to the plan God revealed to me.

As I wrote this book, it was only six years ago that I was given one year to live due to cancer. I am here to show you the five steps I used to become cancer-free just three months after my diagnosis without the use of traditional medical drugs and therapies. It is important for me to share with you though, that because my tumor was in an area where doctors could operate, I did choose to have it removed.

I wrote this book praying that you are given renewed hope as you read. I broke each step down into three sections:

## The Problem

Each symptom has an underlying root. Here we will dig deeper and reveal what the root of each issue is.

## The Pathway

The good news is that every problem has a solution! Here we will uncover what steps we must take to move away from the problem and into the promise.

## The Promise

It's been said that every action has an equal and opposite reaction. Here we will keep our eyes on the prize and focus on the positive changes we are making to our bodies.

In fact, I have learned that cancer in and of itself is not the true problem. Cancer isn't what made me sick. I had been sick for years leading up to it! Cancer was my body's way of sending smoke signals to signify that something was truly wrong in my body. Cancer is a result of the environment that has been created inside of our bodies. I encourage you to really dig your heels in, embrace the changes that you will be implementing and allow yourself to steward your body the way God designed.

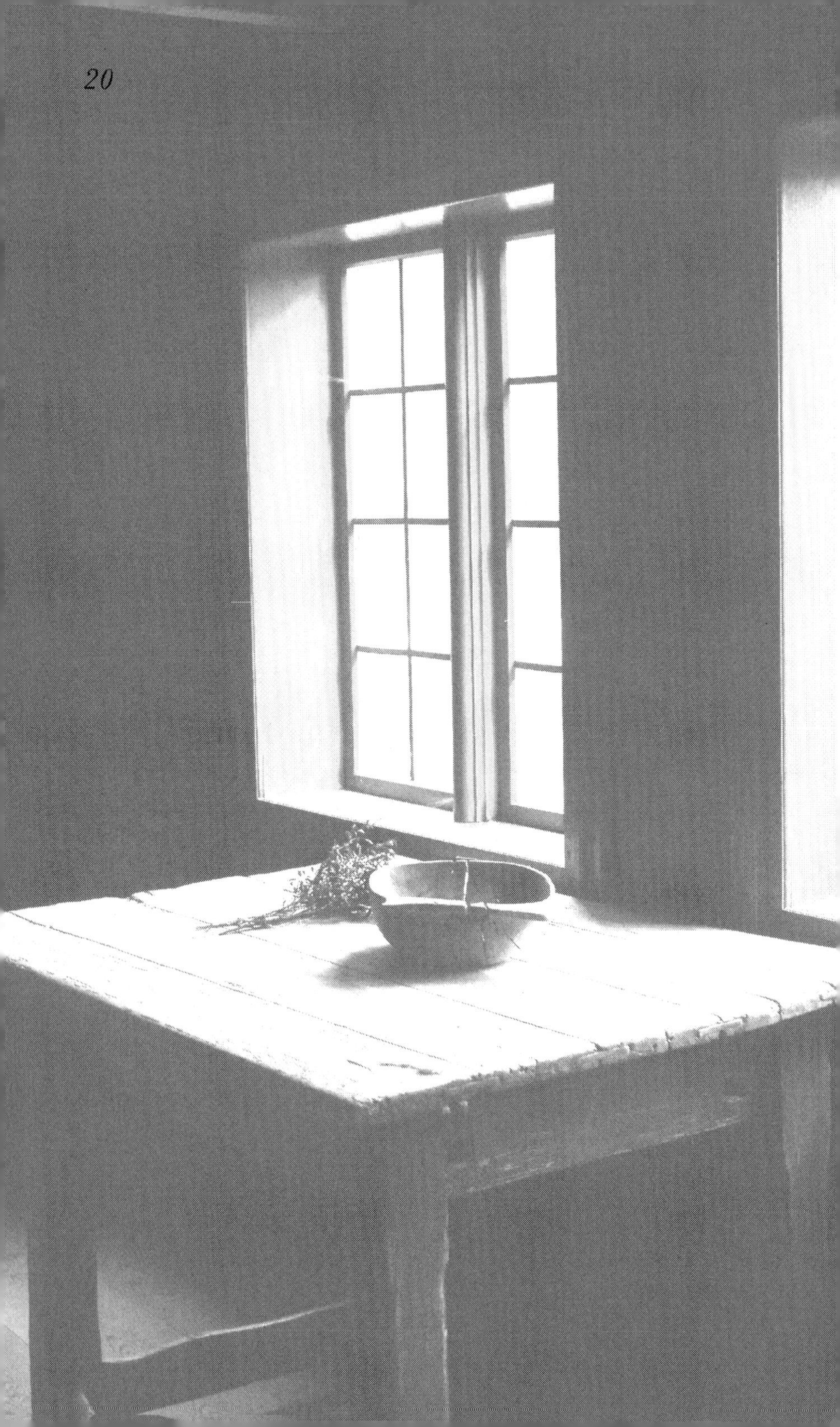

## Understanding The Cancer Components

The further I go in my journey of understanding how to overcome cancer, the more valuable discoveries I make in the process.

When I was diagnosed with cervical cancer in 2012, my story was one where I was incredibly able to be cancer-free in 90 days.

Since that time, I have made it my passion to learn all I can in order to not just stay cancer-free, but also to be as healthy as I can in the rest of my mind and body.

The pursuit has paid off.

In the summer of 2018, I decided (with the encouragement of my physician, Dr. Raymond Hilu) to spend two full weeks getting "re-treated" for any and all potential cancer threats in Marbella, Spain.

While I wasn't diagnosed again with cancer, through routine in-depth blood analysis, Dr. Hilu and I would monitor my blood, and he had some concern that there were some new developments in my body, and, therefore, we decided that I would travel to his clinic in Europe to go through some protocol treatments.

It was completely worth it, and after re-testing following my trip to Spain, my levels are normal and healthy.

In the process of being there, I was able to understand that cancer isn't necessarily a disease. For those of you who would take issue with that statement, I'm not trying to pick a fight.

However, I discovered that cancer is ultimately a result of four main areas:

1) **Diet**
2) **Stress**
3) **Contamination (aka Toxins)**
4) **Genetics**

Rather than simply harping on the negative part of each of these areas, I found the liberating joy of beginning to address each of these areas in a healthy way in order to make a massive difference in my life. One of the main things that I now know is that genetics is actually a very small part in how cancer (and other diseases) take root and grow.

**Think of each of these four areas as a leg on a table.** We want all four legs to be sturdy (healthy) and in as much balance as possible.

*I discovered that cancer is ultimately a result of four main areas.*

This discovery has been amazing for me. In my case of visiting Dr. Hilu, through in-depth blood analysis and consultation, we were able to determine that stress in my life was creating a potential cancer threat in my body.

I'm not going to try and defend why I had been through an extended season of stress but let me say that I am now dealing with it so much better, and it's making a wonderful and positive difference in my health.

In my case, stress was causing issue, but that doesn't mean it's the biggest culprit for everyone. The point though is that in each of the four areas (diet, stress, contamination and genetics) it is possible to identify the root cause(s) of cancer, and other diseases as well.

I want you to know this as you prepare to read my journey of practically how I beat cancer.

My hope and prayer is that it creates a life-giving understanding as to how much of the effect cancer has on us long-term actually is something we can control and help resolve.

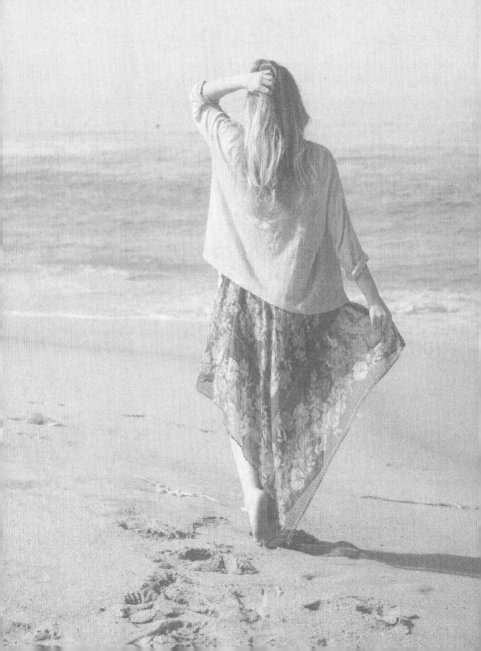

## Step One:

# Renew Your Mind ▶

"Don't copy the behavior and customs of this world, but let God transform you into a new person by changing the way you think. Then you will learn to know God's will for you, which is good and pleasing and perfect."

Romans 12:2

## The Problem

When God formed us, He gave us the innate ability to think for ourselves. He didn't create us to be robots that wander the earth singing His praises day in and day out.

No, He gave us the gift of free will and free thinking. From the moment we are conceived, our brains begin to develop, and we begin forming belief systems based off what we are experiencing.

If we were born to parents who were abusive and lived life in a constant state of fighting, we will more than likely begin to believe that life is a hard battle and that abuse to ourselves and others is normal. If we were born to parents who were attentive and showed unconditional love, we will learn to love others and ourselves the same.

Now, we live in a fallen world. I don't think that there is a single person who has gone through their entire childhood without experiencing some sort of hurt and rejection. Each life experience gives us the opportunity to form thoughts and belief systems.

From a scientific standpoint, every time we have a thought, our brain creates a groove, or pathway if you will, in our brain. Every time we have the same reoccurring thought, the groove gets deeper and deeper into the brain, making it harder and harder to iron out if needed.

If you've lived your entire life thinking that you are a failure or a disappointment, you are going to live as though you are a failure and a disappointment! I could have spent my life allowing my past to dictate my thoughts.

*I'm a divorced woman...no one wants me.*
*I use to work in the strip clubs...I am unclean.*
*I am addicted to sugar...I will never have self-control.*

But thank God we don't have to live that way!

The truth is that many of us are completely unaware of the thoughts that go in and out of our head on a daily basis. A study showed that it's possible we could have up to 60,000 thoughts per day! It also showed that on average, 98% of those thoughts are reoccurring, meaning that you've had them every day for days on end![1]

If you're someone who suffers from "stinkin thinkin," that is a scary statistic!

The good news is that our brain has a distinct ability to be changed and renewed. Your negative thoughts don't have to be permanent!

You can let go of being a victim to your past and your belief systems and take back power and authority over your thought life!

The Bible says to *"be transformed by the renewing of your mind."*[2] Notice that it doesn't say, "Renew your mind," but it says, "renewing." Meaning that it is an ongoing process and not a "one and done" type of experience.

When I was fighting my cancer diagnosis, I had to take my thoughts captive and maximize my mind to it's fullest potential. I knew that if I went into battle

---

1       http://www.jenniferhawthorne.com/articles/change_
your_thoughts.html
2       Romans 12:2

with the mindset of a failure, I would fail. But if I went into it with the mindset of a winner, I could come out victorious!

## The Pathway

When you are battling your own mind, it can be easy to feel overwhelmed and feel as though you do not know where to start. Here is what my process looked like:

*Take Ownership of What You Allow In.* You are the doorkeeper to your own house! Who are you letting into your house (mind)? In today's society, we are inundated with voices from Facebook friends, Instagram influencers, and media outlets! Take an honest look at who your friends are, who you follow and what you are watching. Are these voices bringing you hope or shame? Are they sending you into a spiral of comparison or fear? Take back your ownership and get ruthless when it comes to who has a voice in your head! Unfriend, unfollow and stop those DVR recordings if you have to!

*Meditate on God's Promises.* I knew that once I cleared out who I allowed in my head, I had to fill the vacant space with the promises of God. I set aside time each and every day to be intentional about filling my mind with the Word. I researched every scripture I could about healing and I set my mind on focusing on those promises. I would write them out on giant post cards and stick them on my wall, my mirror, on my fridge, or in my car. Everywhere I went, I had that constant reminder that God heals!

*Use Your Words.* Have you ever seen a toddler throw a tantrum? They kick and scream but they continually get nothing accomplished because they aren't using their words to say what is bothering them. As a mom myself, I would often times have to say, "Use your words!" The same can be true for us. God gave us the gift of speech, and through our words, our worlds are formed. Job 22:28 tells us to *"declare a thing and it will be established."* I took that truth and I ran with it! I made a list of all the promises that God gave me and I continually spoke them over my life. I took the authority that I had in Christ and partnered it with my words. I declared that I was healed, whole and cancer-free!

*If you've lived your entire life thinking that you are a failure or a disappointment, you are going to live as though you are a failure and a disappointment!*

*Check Your Beliefs.* One of the lies that I had to over-come was that cancer had the final say. As I mentioned earlier, we've been conditioned to believe that cancer is incurable. I had to position my thoughts and my mind in alignment with God. Pastor Bill Johnson of Bethel Church says, "I cannot afford to have a thought in my head that is not in His." There is so much power in that statement! The truth is that God is not afraid of cancer! God does not feel intimidated by the presence of it, so, therefore, I refused to allow it to scare me as well. As I researched the truth about cancer, I was floored by the number of people who were able to successfully defeat it without the use of traditional medical methods. As I aligned my belief systems with God, He was faithful to bring people to me who helped me along the journey.

## The Promise

I'll be as straitghforward as possible with you. Renewing your mind might be the single hardest step of this book simply because as humans, we tend to get stuck in our ways.

However, I believe that once you set your mind on becoming a champion, you will see the greatest break-through!

I truly believe that it was because I set my mind on the things of God that I was able to beat cancer as quickly as I did. My life verse is Psalm 103:3, which says, *"He forgives all my sins and he heals all my diseases."* That would include cancer! It gave me such hope to constantly remind myself that God not only forgives us, but He heals us! The Bible is full of promises of health and healing it is our job to take hold of those promises and saturate ourselves in its truth.

▶

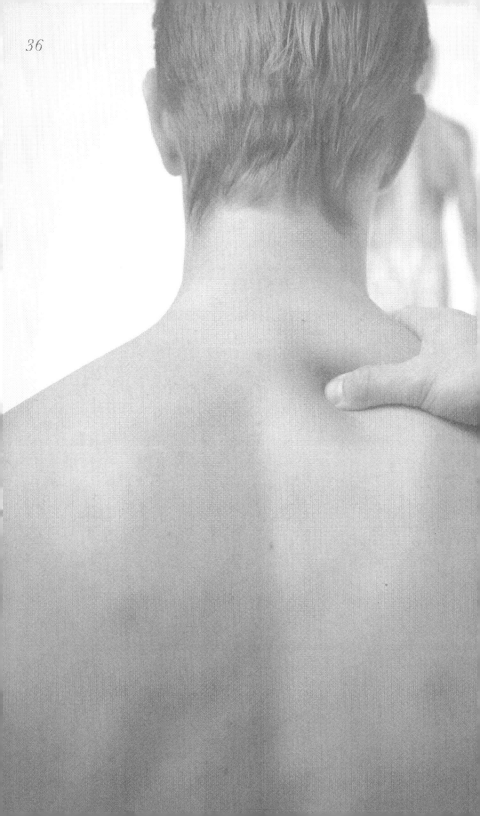

**Step Two:**

# Realign Your Nervous System ▶

*"Light is sown like seed for the righteous, and gladness for the upright in heart."*

*Psalm 97:11*

## The Problem

Most, if not all of us, have been to a chiropractor at least once in our lives. While there are many myths and misleading information out there when it comes to chiropractors, I can say from my own experience that being adjusted is absolutely vital when it comes to living a healthy life.

Not only did it heal things within my body, it began to create a healthy defense mechanism against other disease and illness.

It's that simple.

Chiropractic adjustments focus on realigning the body and primarily the nervous system. Life flows from the nervous system, so when our body is out of alignment, it can block the flow of important nerves and blood flow. For example, I remember my chiropractor telling me that the nerve that innervates to the heart can block up to 65% and the only symptom you may experience is actually a heart attack. That's a scary thought!

When I began going to the chiropractor, I had an x-ray done of my spine and found I had a scoliosis in my L2, L3 and L4 of my lumbar spine. You have cranial and spinal nerves that innervate to specific organs to your body. The spinal nerves that run through the L2, L3 and L4 of the lumbar spines, one of their functions is to innervate to the female and male reproductive system, which includes the cervix for women, which is where I had cancer.

Because my body was out of alignment, my cervix was not receiving the life source from my nervous system that it needed, which is what made it more vulnerable for disease and in my case, cancer.

There are various ways our bodies can be forced out of alignment. Everything from working out, sleeping wrong, bad posture, to sitting, just to name a few, can wreak havoc on our bodies if we are not careful to correct it. With that said, chances are that if you are living and breathing, your body needs to be adjusted! Ideally, you need ongoing corrective (aka "preventative") care, which is really just front-end care to help solve issues before they become major. In most cases though, people go for pain-management care (aka "reactive", which is basically what it sounds like - treatment that attempts to resolve painful problems we may be experiencing.

## The Pathway

It's been said that adjustments can add up to 15 years to your life! If that's not reason enough to start getting adjusted, I don't know what is! Every time you get an adjustment, it helps strengthen and build your immune system, which is essential to helping your body fight disease.[1]

I want to stress the importance of not skipping this step. Many people have become so used to feeling unwell that they have no idea what it feels like to be healthy!

If you had asked me on July 31, 2012 how I felt, I would have replied with an enthusiastic "Great!" It wouldn't have been a lie. I did believe that I felt great. However, the next day, I was diagnosed with cancer. Talk about a mind game! I learned that health is not the absence of symptoms, sickness or disease but the presence of life.

I began to get adjustments 3-4 times a week. I did this for two years, even after my cancer was "gone" because

---

1        https://draxe.com/10-researched-benefits-chiropractic-adjustments/

I believe in the importance of maintenance. After two years, I went down to getting adjusted 1-2 times a week. I still continue to get adjusted every week to this day!

> *Not only did it heal things within my body, it began to create a healthy defense mechanism against other disease and illness.*

Dan Sullivan described chiropractic care by saying, "A chiropractic adjustment influences many aspects of human performance because it removes interference from the brain and central system, allowing the nervous system to perceive and coordinate more efficiently and effectively."[2]

## The Promise

In my journey, I've come to learn that our bodies are fascinating creations that know how to heal themselves when given the proper tools. For example, I suffered from vertigo for three years. Anyone who has experienced it can attest to the fact that it can completely derail your entire day! Would you believe that after suffering for three years, my vertigo was completely gone within

---

2        https://www.facebook.com/Chiropractor.Victor/photo

three adjustments? Three years worth of suffering were completely alleviated in just three visits! Amazing!

As I said, when I first began going to my chiropractor, I had no idea how bad I actually felt until I began to see a difference after a few adjustments. The good news is that when your spine is aligned the way God created and intended, it is built to last!

▶

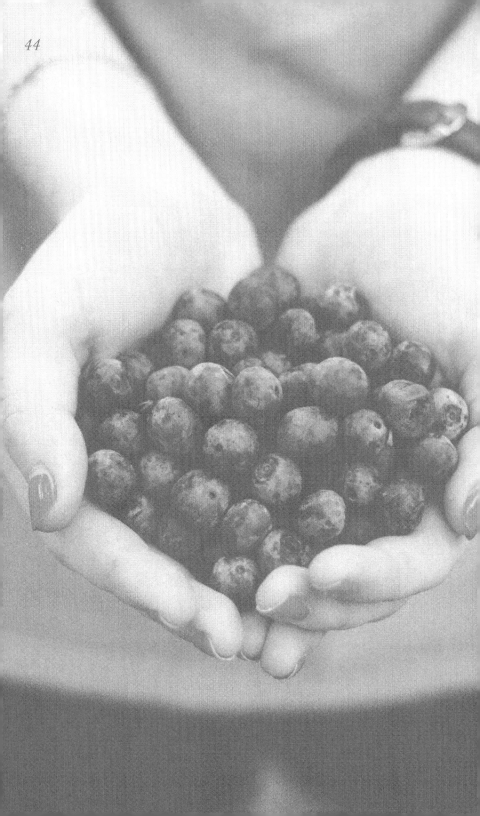

Step Three:

# Revitalize Your Eating ▶

"It is written, 'Man shall not live by bread alone, but by every word that proceeds from the mouth of God.' "

Matthew 4:4

## The Problem

**DIET.** It's a word that society has taught us to resent because with it comes visions of dry rice cakes, chalky protein powders and drawn out walks on the treadmill.

It always breaks my heart to hear people say they hate eating healthy because I truly believe we were created and designed to love the food God created for us.

The problem is that the food industry has loaded our "food" with chemicals and sugars, which make our brain become dependent on them.

**Did you know that the acronym for the Standard American Diet is "SAD"? It is just that – It's SAD!** The standard American diet is, quite frankly, a complete sham. Those at the top are not teaching people how to properly nourish our bodies, but instead, they are encouraging us to poison our bodies!

The standard American diet is filled with processed meat, dairy, unhealthy fats, and sugar! Research studies have found potential links between the standard

American diet and risks of the following diseases and
conditions:
- Muscle loss
- Acne
- Increased rick for Alzheimer's and dementia
- Breast cancer
- Increased levels of IGF-1, a growth hormone
  associated with cancer risk
- Thicker carotid arteries
- High cholesterol
- Increased absorption of endotoxins
- Enlarged prostate and heart attacks
- Increased free radicals
- Heart disease
- Unhealthy inflammation and oxidation
- Greater risk of inflammatory bowel disease
- Reduction of inner blood vessel lining function
- Declining kidney function
- Lower back problems
- Worsening of lung function and asthma control
- Greater risk of pancreatic cancer
- Greater risk of preterm delivery
- Greater risk for prostate cancer
- Obesity
- Small stools
- Decreased sex drive

- Increased rick of autism and cancer in children
- Increased risk of childhood diabetes
- Traces of toxic waste in breast milk[1]

If that list doesn't want to make you run to your nearest juice bar, I don't know what will! As we can see, our eating habits in America have taken a drastic turn from what God intended our diets to be. Even our so-called "health foods" like low-carb yogurts and protein bars are bursting with chemicals, sugars, and synthetic materials. Our bodies, as brilliant as they are, simply do not know how to process chemicals. So, they in turn get stored in our organs and muscles, which then wreaks havoc on everything from our brain to our bones.

To make matters worse, GMOs have now taken precedence in our foods. GMO stands for "Genetically Modified Organism." To simplify, it is a plant, animal, microorganism, or other organism whose genetic makeup has been modified using recombinant DNA methods like gene modification or transgenic technology.[2]

---

1        https://nutritionfacts.org/topics/standard-american-diet/

2        https://www.nongmoproject.org/gmo-facts/

What this means is that even our most basic food needs, like fruits and vegetables, are now being tampered with and manipulated! Most of the produce at your local grocery store isn't even real produce anymore. It could look like a vegetable and taste like a vegetable, but it is not a vegetable. It is a science experiment and we are the guinea pigs that they are testing it on.

Sugar has also become a common culprit that is the cause of sickness and disease. Food manufacturers are loading our everyday foods with hidden sugars.

It's been studied that the average American will consume 150 pounds of sugar a year![3] Some people think that they can avoid sugar by just looking for the word "sugar" on food labels, but food companies actually have sixty-one different names for sugar![4] Sixty-one!

**For many people, sugar is one of the hardest addictions that they will ever have to beat.** However, it is one of the most dangerous substances in our foods, in my opinion. It is highly addictive, eight times more so than cocaine! In addition, it causes

3        https://www.sharecare.com/health/carbohydrates/sugar-consume-every-year
4        http://sugarscience.ucsf.edu/hidden-in-plain-sight/#. WWaRUdPyto4

weight gain, depression, accelerated aging, skin dullness, and inflammation that is linked to numerous diseases, including cancer.

## The Pathway

Next to renewing our mind, this step may be one of the most crucial when it comes to fighting disease! What you feed, grows. If we are feeding our bodies with chemicals and toxins, disease and bacteria will grow inside of us. However, if we are nourishing our bodies with organic fruits, vegetables, and grass-fed and finished meats, life abounds.

As I researched the correlation between food and cancer, I immediately decided to revamp my diet. I eliminated all sugar (including honey and maple syrup), caffeine, grains, gluten, alcohol, and most dairy products.

The dairy that I did eat was very limited and was only organic, raw dairy. My diet primarily consisted of fresh vegetable juice, veggies, healthy fats, and some lean proteins like turkey and some wild-caught fish. I alternated between two juices every day. My first juice was eight ounces total of red cabbage, kale, romaine lettuce, green bell pepper, swiss chard, and lemon. The second juice was eight ounces of ¼ green apple and carrots. I alternated between the two for a total of thirteen times a day. I was also advised to eat a cup of fresh okra every day because of its powerful cancer-fighter properties, and because it is loaded with antioxidants. I also had one whole beet three times a week while incorporating the Budwig Protocol (which can be found in the resources at the end of this book).

The first step in nourishing your body is to flood it with micronutrients. Micronutrients are going to be vitamins and minerals that can only be found in living foods.

As I mentioned before, I went into this battle with the mindset of a champion, so my approach to this was absolutely intense and non-compromising! I invested in a juicer and I began juicing thirteen times a day. I went through three juicers in just a matter of one year.

Extreme? Maybe. **But the fact is that when I changed my diet and replaced the things wreaking havoc in my body with foods that carried life, I knew it was working because three months later there were no more signs of cancer.**

Did you hear what I just said? **After being given only a year to live, I was cancer-free in just three months!**

Now, even though I was juicing, I wasn't on a fully liquid diet. I still needed to be intentional in giving my body other nutrients such as fiber and protein.

Many sources with tell you that you should be getting at least 20 grams of fiber per day, but I would aim for as much as 40-50. The reason for this is that fiber is going to be what cleans out your gut and digestive track, which is where bacteria tends to hide and make room for disease.

I always recommend getting fiber from natural sources likes fruits, vegetables, flax seeds, beans, legumes or chia seeds. However, hitting 50 grams can be hard. You can find a good fiber supplement at your local health food store to help you hit your needed intake.

I personally use a supplement called "Everybody's Fiber" by Nature's Sunshine. Be sure to check the ingredients and steer clear of any that have any added sugars!

When it comes to protein, this can be another tricky road to navigate. Sadly, many of our protein sources have been manipulated as well. Animals are now being fed GMO food sources, like corn, on a daily basis. You've heard the saying "You are what you eat." Well, I like to say, "You are what your food eats!"

You can be doing all the right things by stripping your diet of harmful chemicals, but if you are eating generic chicken or beef, you are only undoing all of your hard work.

**The first step in nourishing your body is to flood it with micronutrients.**

When I began switching to organic products, I knew that eating organic grass-fed and finished meats was important for my health. (If you are unable to afford all organic products, I always recommend first getting organic meats before you switch to organic fruits and vegetables.)

Be sure to find a good fruit and vegetable wash to help wash off those pesticides. Research "The Dirty Dozen" to find which fruits and vegetables have higher levels of pesticides and require more cleaning.

Finding quality meats may require a little digging, but it is so worth it! I always recommend buying from your local farmer because it not only helps support farmers who raise their animals humanely, but most local farmers do not use hormones or antibiotics!

If you cannot find a local farmer near you, it is important to be sure you are buying the right organic meats at your local grocer. Now, marketing has become tricky and is geared towards tricking you into making you believe you are buying healthier options than you are!

For example, many companies use the word "Organic," however, organic-certified chickens can still be raised in terrible living conditions. The key words to look for are Animal Welfare Approved, Certified Humane or the Global Animal Partnership.[5]

Another source of protein to be cautious when buying is eggs. Eggs, out of any other protein source, have the most hormones and antibiotics pumped into them! Again, it is best to purchase from a local, humane farmer when buying. However, if you must go the store bought route, always opt for eggs that are certified organic, pasture-raised, and are high in Omega-3s and DHAs,

5       https://foodbabe.com/2016/03/28/truth-chickens-raised-will-disgust-eating/

and as an additional preference, I like to get the ones that are soy-free.

### One of the most healing substances God has given us is water!

Water does everything from help purify our bloodstreams, to detoxing our organs to flushing out fat! Many of us do not get anywhere near the amount of water we need to be drinking a day. A good rule of thumb is to drink half of your body weight in ounces. I personally aim for a gallon every day.

A vitally important key to maintaining good health is adding supplements to our diets. Our foods naturally have vitamins and minerals in them, but because of technology and changes in our soil, our food has nowhere near the same potency of vitamins that it had even fifty years ago! With that said, it is important that we are giving our bodies the support it needs with supplements.

If you walk into any health food store, you will be bombarded with aisles upon aisles of supplements to choose from! It is easy to be overwhelmed and confused when it comes to which ones your body needs.

I highly suggest finding a holistic doctor in your area who can test your food allergies (called IgG testing) as well as provide a blood-spot metabolic test. This will help diagnose what foods are reactive in your body as well as what vitamins and minerals your body needs to thrive. That will help you immensely in trying to narrow down which ones you need.

**Here are my top supplements that I recommend:**

**Indole-3-Carbinol:** *This may be one of the most important supplements when it comes to fighting cancer, specifically hormone cancers.* It has a variety of different benefits including promoting cancerous cell death, increasing antioxidant activity as well as detoxing the body. It also helps eliminate excess estrogen stored in the body, which can be the culprit to cancers including breast and cervical cancer.[6]

**Probiotics:** Our gut is often referred to as the "second brain," so it is important that we are doing everything we can to keep our gut healthy! Probiotics help keep our gut regular as well as help with mood swings, digestion, vitamin absorbency, and also helps

---

6    https://www.naturessunshine.com/us/product/indole-3-carbinol-60-caps/1506/

strengthen our immune system. Many times, our natural probiotics are killed or weakened due to sugar, medications, antibiotics, NSAIDs, diets with excessive grains, processed foods, and stress! Because of this, we should be taking a probiotic.

**Food and Pancreatic Enzymes:** An enzyme supplement should be taken at every meal to help us break down and absorb nutrients! Food enzymes can help aid everything from digestive disorders, acid reflux, liver disease, iron deficiency, slow metabolism, and leaky gut.

**Curcumin:** Curcumin (more commonly known as turmeric) is a powerful herb that helps greatly reduce inflammation in the body! Inflammation is a leading cause of disease for many Americans and can be easily eliminated with the proper use of turmeric. Be sure to find one that also has black pepper extract in it because it helps increase the absorbency by up to 2000%.

**Methyl B12+Folate:** B12 is essential for a healthy central nervous system. It helps benefit everything from your heart, immune system, skin, hair, digestion, and mood! I recommend finding a liquid methyl B12 supplement or a B12 injection so that it can bypass the digestive system and go straight into your blood stream.

It can also be found in most animal products such as meat, fish, liver, and eggs.

**Omega-3:** Omega-3 Fatty Acids are lifesavers when it comes to treating conditions like asthma, depression, fetus development, ADHA, as well as Alzheimer's, dementia, and cancer. They also help lower inflammation in the body and aid in absorbing vital nutrients and minerals.

**Vitamin D3:** The majority of our society is extremely deficient in Vitamin D3. Vitamin D3 is naturally produced in our bodies when we are in the sun without the use of sunscreen. It helps fight disease, boosts your immune system, alleviates depression, promotes weight loss, and helps with absorption of calcium and phosphorous.

**Whole Food Multivitamin:** A solid, whole food multivitamin is a great way to help replenish your body with vitamins and minerals. For athletes or those on a limited diet, it can be hard to get all the nutrients that your body needs. The reason I am recommending investing in a whole food multivitamin as opposed to a generic one is that the generic ones are filled with synthetic fillers. They have also been processed, and as we know, we want as few processed substances going into our bodies as possible! Two of my favorite multi-vitamins are "Revive" sold by Uncorked Wellness and "Super Trio" by Nature's Sunshine.

**Berberine IR:** This is one of my favorite supplements because I believe that just about anyone can benefit from this! Berberine IR is great for balancing blood sugar and glucose levels so that your cells are able to then work and support each other. Diabetes is out of control and is continuing to grow, but that is a whole other book I could write about!

**Magnesium:** The role that Magnesium plays in our bodies is enormous. In the process of overcoming cancer, I discovered that it is considered the most important mineral in our body.

## The Promise

The Apostle Paul tells us in Romans to offer our bodies as a living sacrifice as an act of worship. We cannot offer a dead body as a sacrifice! As I went through this journey, I learned the importance of viewing our bodies as the temple that God created it to be. In the

Old Testament, before anyone could even enter into the temple, they had to go through a strict regimen to be declared clean. God has only ever wanted the best to enter His temple! Now, we no longer go to a temple to worship but instead we have become the temple of God. When we honor God with our bodies, we get to reap the rewards!

I realize that changing our diets can be hard for many, especially if you are accustomed to eating processed food and sugary treats. In this case, I can't stress enough the importance of finding what your Why is. In the moments when I found myself being tempted to eat food that was not healthy for me, I had to ask myself, "Will this food produce death or life?" I had to make the decision that my family, health, and life were worth far more than any unhealthy food could provide for me.

▶

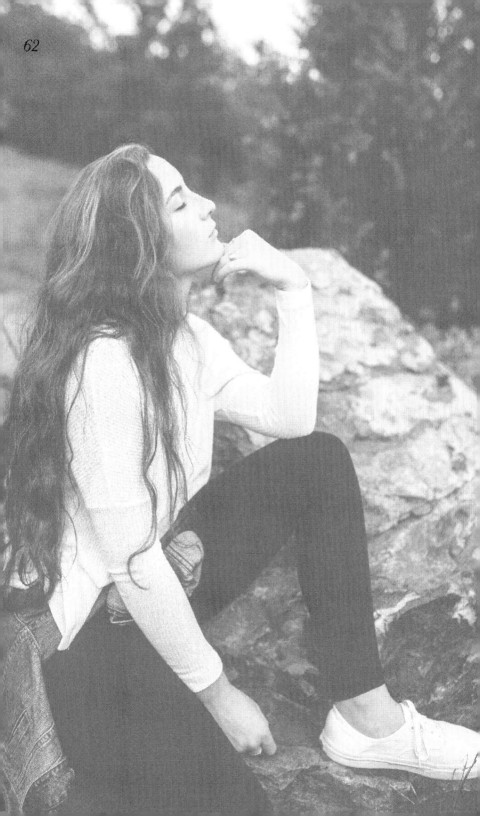

**Step Four:**

# Restore Your Energy ▶

"The Spirit of God has made me, and the breath of the Almighty gives me life."

Job 33:4

## The Problem

The problem with this step is short and simple: People can be lazy and don't like to workout. Our bodies were designed to be active!

Hundreds of years ago, people didn't need to workout because their lives kept them active and healthy! They didn't have cars to get them to and from work or grocery stores to hunt and prepare their food for them. They had to do it all themselves.

Now, we hardly have to use our bodies for any physical labor other than getting up from our computers to walk five feet to the coffee machine!

It's common for people to think that they only have to workout if they want to lose weight. While weight loss can be an added bonus, that is only one of many benefits to exercise. **Here's what happens to our bodies when we choose to not exercise:**

- Increased blood pressure
- Weight gain

- Loss of bone density
- Increased risk of osteoporosis
- Decreased energy
- Increased risk of depression and low self-esteem
- Increased risk for diabetes
- Spike in unhealthy food cravings
- Risk for insomnia
- Spike in stress levels
- Causes unbalanced hormones
- Decreased sex drive
- Decrease in oxygen levels

## The Pathway

I learned in my journey that cancer cannot survive in an oxygenated environment! With that said, an exercised body is an oxygenated body! At the beginning of my cancer journey, I didn't have all the energy that I was used to having. There were days when I felt weak, but I made it a priority to move my body in one way or another. I committed to exercising at least three days a week until I could get my energy built up.

Every body is different so everyone is going to have a different workout preference. My best piece of advice for finding what works for your body is to find out what blood type you are. I am personally a type AB. This means that I benefit from a mix of calming exercise as well as intense exercises such as cardio and weight lifting.

My energy was low starting out, so I incorporated a lot of yoga, stretching, and walking. These low-impact workouts are great for helping balance hormones! I also was able to incorporate step one (Renew your Mind) into my walks because I turned them into prayer walks!

As my energy increased, I was able to begin to incorporate light weight lifting and cardio.

**I've found that many women have an irrational fear when it comes to weight lifting because they think that it will make them bulky.**

However, nothing is further from the truth! Weight lifting has many benefits including maintaining bone density and balancing your hormones. It also helps flush out any toxins that are being stored in our muscles!

I eventually was able to begin one of my favorite types of workouts: HIIT training. HIIT stands for High Intensity Interval Training. HIIT utilizes the strength of your heart and helps promote fast weight loss and toxin removal. An example of a common HIIT practice is done with running, where you run as fast as you can for 1 minute and then walk for 2 minutes. You repeat for a total of 15 minutes. Or, you can run in place for 20 seonds and rest for 20 seconds, and repeat for 12 minutes.

This type of workout is often utilized by a lot of athletes because of its ability to build endurance, burn fat while preserving muscle as well as increase overall energy. I gained a lot of knowledge from a program called Max T-3 by Living where they designed twelve-minute HIIT workouts that any person can complete. I truly believe that despite who you are, where you're from, or what your blood type is that everyone can benefit from HIIT workouts because of it's unique ability to challenge and strengthen the body as well as detox and reshape it.

I also incorporated a lot of what is called "grounding" into my lifestyle. Now, I know that this may seem a little strange to some, but grounding has been scientifically proven to help increase the overall quality of life!

You see, the earth is magnetic and has electrical fields running all throughout it. Likewise, our bodies have an electrical currency as well! Ages ago, humanity used to walk barefoot, sleep on the ground, and in general have more physical contact with the earth.

> *It's common for people to think that they only have to workout if they want to lose weight.*

Since we've progressed, it is very rare for any of us to be outside without shoes on! Studies have shown that being in direct contact with the ground, whether it's dirt, grass, sand, or pools of water, have an enormous impact on our body's ability to function.

One study showed that "It can help restore and stabilize the bioelectrical circuitry that governs your physiology and organs, harmonize your basic biological rhythms, boost self-healing mechanisms, reduce inflammation and pain, and improve your sleep and feeling of calmness."[1]

As long as it wasn't down pouring or snowing, I was consistent about getting my grounding time in. I spent at least twenty minutes a day, barefoot in the dirt and grass,

---

1       https://heartmdinstitute.com/alternative-medicine/what-is-earthing-or-grounding/

preferably damp. Another bonus to this was that I was able to also soak up the sunrays, which helps pump our bodies with Vitamin D as well as balance our melatonin levels. I also used this time to maximize my mind and mediate on the promises of God.

## The Promise

**The benefits of exercise far outweigh the burden of having to just do it!** Just adding 30 minutes of exercise to your routine 3-5 days a week will:
  • Improve sleep quality
  • Promote weight loss
  • Help balance blood sugar
  • Improve memory
  • Fight disease
  • Increase circulation
  • Balance hormones
  • Alleviate depression
  • Prevent injury
  • Increase life span
  • Reduce your risk of heart disease
  • Reduce stress

Exercise is just another way that we are able to offer our bodies to God as an act of worship. I encourage you to find a workout that you enjoy doing and look forward to! I can almost guarantee that you will not regret it!

▶

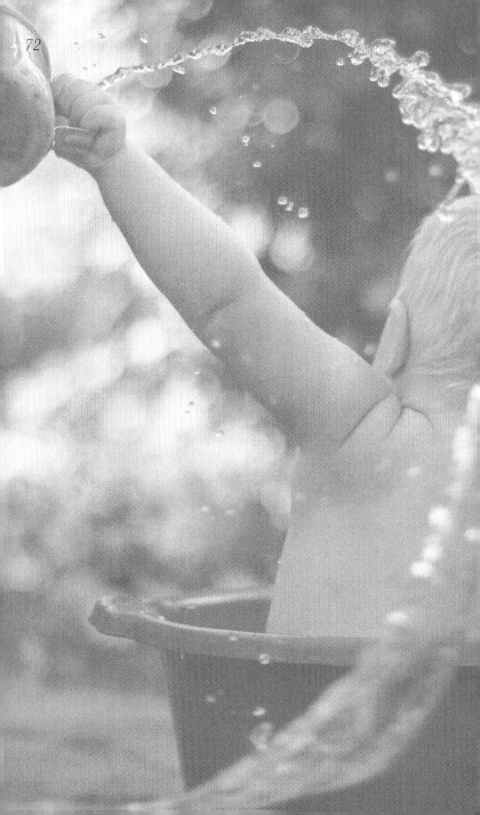

**Step Five:**

# Remove Your Toxicity ▶

*"Beloved, I pray that in all respects you may prosper and be in good health, just as your soul prospers."*

*3 John 1:2*

## The Problem

Toxins are everywhere. They are in the air we breathe, the cleaning products we use, the food we eat, and the beauty products we slather on ourselves, just to name a few.

I will say right off the bat that it is next to impossible to be able to fully avoid taking in toxins! To do so, we would have to live in a secluded area without any contact with the modern world, and let's face it: that sounds real boring!

The scary part is that many of us have no idea the amount of chemicals that we are coming across on a daily basis. For example, our skin is the largest organ on our bodies and everything we put on our skin gets absorbed and pushed into our blood stream.

Being a woman, I can say that I enjoy nice products that smell good! But…

Every day I was slathering on perfume laden lotions without any idea the harm that it was causing to my body! They had toxic chemicals like benzaldehyde, camphor, ethyl acetate, benzyl acetate, linalool, acetone, aluminum, lauryl sulfate, and methylene chloride. These have been found to cause dizziness, nausea, drowsiness, irritation to throat, eyes, skin, and lungs, kidney damage, headaches, cancers, and other diseases!

*Every day I was slathering on perfume laden lotions without any idea the harm that it was causing to my body!*

Our cleaning products that we use are also bombarded with toxic chemicals! Most of us clean with the hopes of preventing harmful bacteria from being able to harm us, yet we are just fixing that problem with another problem!

**A study found that the average household has as many as sixty-two harmful chemicals!** These chemicals have been linked to diseases such as asthma, cancers, reproductive disorders, hormone disruption, and neurotoxicity.[1]

---

1       https://experiencelife.com/article/8-hidden-toxins-whats-lurking-in-your-cleaning-products/

We also are inhaling chemicals on a daily basis. Everything from pollution in the air to harmful chemicals in air fresheners can have a dramatic effect on our bodies and have been linked to serious health effects, such as cancer, birth defects, immediate death, or other serious illnesses.[2]

It's no wonder why millions of Americans are finding themselves sick, depressed and hopeless! Thankfully, there is always a solution.

## The Pathway

When I became sick, my health coach came into my house and raided everything from my kitchen cabinets and fridge to my makeup bag and beauty products! It was a shock, to say the least, to see so many things get thrown into a giant trash bag!

When it came to food products, if it had an ingredient in it that we couldn't pronounce, we tossed it! *If it had a longer shelf life than me, it was gone!* A good rule of thumb is to eat foods that only have 5 ingredients or less. Anything that has a long list of ingredients is more than likely not natural and is not

2        https://www3.epa.gov/airtoxics/3_90_023.html

going to bring healing to your body! I always say, "If mold won't eat it, you shouldn't eat it."

I know that many women may have a hard time parting ways with their favorite cosmetics or beauty products. It's understandable because we tend to stick with what we know and love. However, as I began this journey, I was amazed at all the healthy, organic cosmetic and beauty alternatives out there! I will go into further detail on this later in the chapter.

The air we breathe is something that we may not have a lot of control over, however, we are able to control what scents we bring into our house. Many people are accustomed to using air fresheners in their homes and cars. Everything from candles, wall units, to bathroom sprays are common household products, but they come with a costly price! Many of them are filled with a harmful chemical called Phthalates. Here is a quote from the Natural Resources Defense Counsel:

"Phthalates are hormone-disrupting chemicals that can be particularly dangerous for young children and unborn babies. Exposure to phthalates can affect testosterone levels and lead to reproductive abnormalities, including abnormal genitalia and reduced sperm production. The State of California notes that five types of phthalates -- including one that we found in air freshener products -- are 'known to cause birth defects or reproductive harm.'"[3]

> *I can't help but wonder if the reason we are seeing an increase in birth defects, infertility, and tragic pregnancies has to do with the chemicals in the air we are inhaling.*

A few years ago, we had someone come out and replace our air filters. After he was finished, he asked if I burned candles often. I proudly said, "Yes!" I loved having yummy scented candles around the house and had at least one in every room! He showed me the air filters that he took out and they were completely jet-black. He said, "I could tell because all the candle residue gets stuck in the filters."

Seeing how the candles affected the air filters forced me to open my eyes to the truth of what I was subjecting my family and myself to inhale on a daily basis. If you

---

3    http://healthwyze.org/reports/184-how-air-fresheners-are-killing-you

think about it, our lungs and liver are our God-given filter system. If the candles were causing that much damage to our AC vents, what was it doing inside of me?

## The Alternatives

As I said, it is next to impossible to be able to avoid all the toxins in our world, but you are able to at least limit and manage them.

**Makeup:** Parting ways with our favorite makeup products can be painful! Trust me, I know! However, I had to weigh the pros and cons and I came to the realization that risking my health for a little makeup coverage just wasn't worth it! I was able to find an amazing makeup artist and aesthetician that actually makes my products for me using only clean ingredients. Everything from my cleansers and moisturizers to my foundation and mascara is tailored made. If you do your research, you can find good clean makeup and beauty products that are free of harmful chemicals! Many times, your local health food store will carry clean makeup and body products.

**Deodorant:** Our common deodorants are filled with cancer causing chemicals, primarily aluminum.

Making your own deodorant is actually fairly easy to do from home, as well as inexpensive. There are also some great deodorant brands like Schmidts and Primal Paste that have effective and natural ingredients.

**Air Fresheners:** Since I favor products that air on the side of nature, I have found that high quality essential oils can be of great use in the home. They can be diffused to help eliminate odors and even used in place of cleaning products around the home.

**Cleaning Products:** My motto is: the simpler, the better! There are many great blogs that have ideas for natural cleaning products to use. I have learned to clean with normal, everyday products like baking soda, apple cider vinegar, and good quality essential oils.

**Cooking Ware:** Most of our modern day cookware is also extremely toxic. Nonstick cookware is loaded with chemicals that can affect everything from your hormones to your sleep cycles! I switched all my cookware and bakeware to waterless stainless steel and glass, and made sure there was no lead in the glass. I understand good cookware is often expensive, but cast-iron made in the USA is fantastic (a good, reputable company is Lodge) . I also got rid of all my plastic Tupperware and switched to glass because the plastic also has harmful chemicals that get saturated in your food when used for storage. I found that Costco has the more affordable glass Tupperware set. I also recommend swapping out aluminum foil for unbleached parchment paper. Once again, the aluminum foil has harmful chemicals that leach into our food, especially when heated.

**Microwave:** In 1946, a man by the name of Percy Spencer invented the microwave. They quickly became the hottest kitchen appliance and eventually found their way into every kitchen. People loved the convenience of having food go from cold to hot in a mere 60 seconds. For years, I also used a microwave thinking that it benefited my life. However, I soon discovered that microwaves may be one of the most dangerous appliances found in the modern home. One of the reasons is because it not only uses radiation to heat your food, it also causes most of the nutrients in your food to die off.[4] I highly recommend investing in a toaster oven or convection oven and opting for that in place of a microwave.

**Detox Options**

---

4        https://www.globalhealingcenter.com/natural-health/
why-you-should-never-microwave-your-food/

**Coffee Enemas:** Since we are constantly being bombarded with toxins, I always recommend finding ways to detox your system as well. For myself, I began doing coffee enemas regularly. Coffee enemas are a great detoxification for the liver. The way it works is the coffee is absorbed into your system and goes directly to the liver where it becomes a very strong toxin eliminator. It causes the liver to produce more bile (which contains processed toxins) and moves bile out towards the small intestine for elimination. It also helps the body produce glutathione, which is powerful when it comes to fighting cancer. Glutathione is a strong antioxidant, which is concentrated in the liver but found in every cell of the body. Its job is to search out and destroy anything that would pose a threat such as heavy metals, toxins, and free radicals. I did these up to eight times a day for a few months because I had cancer and needed to detox. Once my body became less toxic, I went down to two times a week for the next year and a half.

**Infrared Saunas:** Infrared saunas are a great way to sweat out toxins that are stored in your body! In addition, infared is one of the vest ways to eliminate heavy metals from the body. They work by using heat and light to help detoxify, as well as relax the body. Heat therapies, such as saunas, have been around for hundreds of years dating back to the Native Americans. Sweating is one of the best things you can do for your body! It helps regulate blood flow, flushes out the lymphatic system, reduces inflammation, and clears skin, just to name a few. Infrared saunas are different than regular saunas because they use light technology to raise your body temperature, and much like having a fever, they make you sweat. They also awaken and reactivate your cells. When I went to the sauna, I would sit in it for sixty minutes, three to five days a week. Be sure to refer to your health care provider for what is safe for you.

**Intravenous Heavy Metal Pushes:** Our bodies have a tendency to have a collection of heavy metals stored inside. Just a few of the ways we come into contact with heavy metals on a daily basis is through cookware, fireworks, baking powder, antiperspirants, toothpaste, processed dairy, cans, seafood, and dentures. (As a side note, I actually had my mercury fillings removed and replaced with composite material that is non-toxic. Be sure to find a dentist who uses safe practices when removing and replacing mercury fillings). Heavy metals are extremely toxic to our bodies and as you can see, they are hard to avoid! The intravenous heavy metal pushes flooded my system with different vitamins and minerals that helped push those heavy metals out. This detox process may have been the single most painful process. I remember being so sick from the detox that I was hardly able to move or do anything! However, the results were worth the pain.

**Intravenous Vitamin C:** I also incorporated intravenous Vitamin C into my regimen. You may be asking yourself why this was necessary when I could have easily just taken a Vitamin C supplement. When Vitamin C is taken orally, it acts as an anti-oxidant, which is means it's job is to fight free radicals. However, cancer cells actually have a thick protein wall called fibrin built around them because its main goal is to survive and grow. Many nutrients are unable to break into the wall, making it hard for the cancer cells to ever be killed off. So when taken orally, Vitamin C is unable to actually penetrate the cancer cells. When Vitamin C is taken intravenously, it acts as a pro-oxidant. The cancer cells then are tricked into letting the Vitamin C go through its walls and into the cell, which in turn then kills the cancer cells. Can I get a Hallelujah on that one?! I did this procedure three times a week for the first 18 months of my regimen.

**Candida Cleanse:** A common condition many Americans have is yeast overgrowth. Yeast overgrowth happens when the body is overloaded with sugar and it cannot be broken down. It is often the cause of sickness and diseases such as irritable bowel syndrome, stomach pain and cramps, insomnia, chronic UTIs, and mood swings. Diet will many times help significantly decrease candida overgrowth when you eliminate all sources of sugar, grains and gluten. I would recommend asking your naturopath doctor to order a home fecal test to find out if you have candida overgrowth. This will help determine which strand(s) of candida you actually have and will be efficient when choosing which candida detox would be best for you.

**Plants:** We should also be eliminating toxins in our air when possible. One of my favorite ways to detox the air is by buying fresh, indoor plants! Plants are God's natural air cleaners! NASA actually performed a study on the benefits of having indoor plants, and they found that indoor plants made a significant impact on chemical reduction, primarily with chemicals like trichloroethylene and formaldehyde.[5] Some great indoor plant options are Peace Lilies and Spider Plants.

**Salt Lamps:** Himalayan Salt Lamps have also grown in popularity over the recent years due to their health benefits. Dr. Josh Axe explains how they work the best:

---

5        http://butternutrition.com/detoxifying-indoor-plants-air-filters/

"Salt is hygroscopic, which means it attracts water molecules to itself. Being the big hunk of salt that it is, a Himalayan salt lamp is believed to work by attracting the water molecules. This water vapor can also carry **indoor air pollutants** like mold, bacteria and allergens. Once the water vapor comes in contact with the salt lamp, the pollutants are believed to remain trapped in the salt. Since the lamp is heated, the salt dries out and is able to continue the cycle of attracting water vapor and pollutants, releasing the water vapor back into the air but holding on to the health-hazardous pollutants."[6]

Many people report feeling relief from allergies and grogginess as well as an increase in sleep quality, energy, and mood! Be sure to do your research and invest in a real salt lamp, as there are many fake ones on the market.

6    https://draxe.com/himalayan-salt-lamp/

## The Promise

I quickly learned that I can not live as a control freak and allow myself to become stressed out over things that are beyond my ability to change. However, I learned the importance in stewarding what I could change. This step can be uncomfortable because many of us have grown up using these everyday products, so it can feel like unchartered territory.

The truth is, we are responsible for stewarding and caring for the bodies that have been entrusted to us. In the Old Testament, the temple was never allowed to be polluted and dirtied because the Spirit of God resided within.

The same is true for our bodies. We should be intentionally taking inventory of what we are allowing into our bodies and what needs to be released and cleaned out so that we can operate to our fullest, God-given potential.

▶

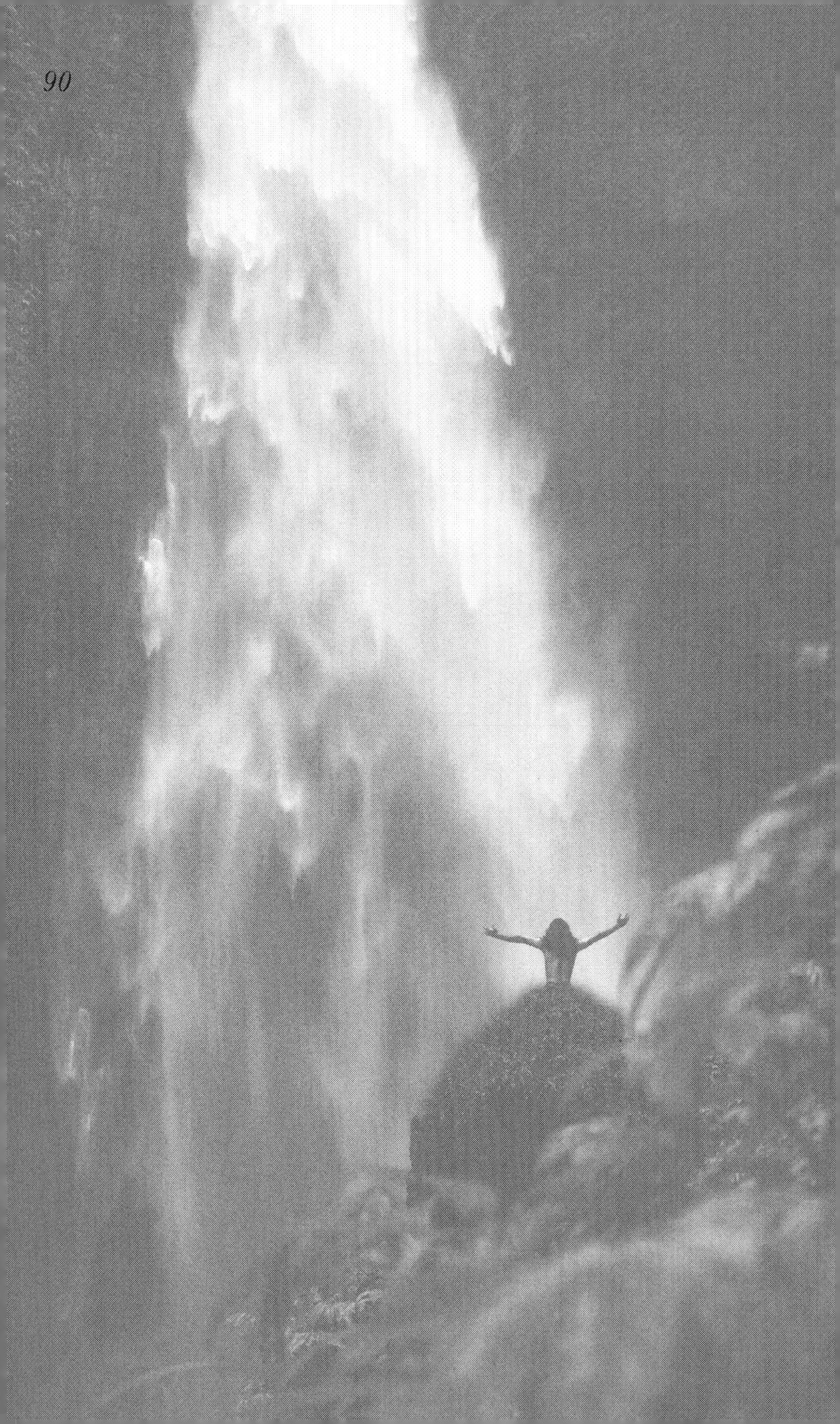

## Bonus:

# My Specialized Protocols ▶

*"Behold, I am doing a new thing! Now it springs forth; do you not perceive and know it and will you not give heed to it? I will even make a way in the wilderness and rivers in the desert."*

*Isaiah 43:19*

## Let me be clear.

The protocols and treatments that I'm about to share with you were all done with the oversight and/or supervision of trained medical professionals.

In other words, it's not something to launch into on your own.

These protocols are, unfortunately, currently not-so-common in the United States. However, without a doubt, they are the driving force behind not only my journey of overcoming cancer, but countless others as well. I can say firsthand that they work in destroying cancer.

Because I get asked almost daily what were the protocols I used/went through, I wanted to be able to share them with you.

I'd like to thank Dr. Raymond Hilu, from Clinica Hilu in Marbella, Spain (clinicahilu.com) for allowing me to use his explanations for the majority of the protocol descriptions, and for his life-saving influence in my life.

## BIOCATALYTIC OXYGENATION

By inhaling oxygenation catalysts, such as those produced by plants, like oxygen at the time of photosynthesis, the biocatalyst plays a role of "supertransmitter" in oxygen metabolism. It is useful for chronic coughing, fatigue, nervousness, forgetfulness, anorexia, bulimia, heart disturbances, cardiovascular problems, circulation, etc.

The cells undergoing biocatalytic oxygenation resist +25% above the normal average.

The air around is composed of 21% oxygen. When we breathe, air enters the airways to the alveoli, where gas exchange occurs and oxygen from the air diffuses through the blood. In the blood, over 95% of oxygen attaches to hemoglobin, a major protein in red blood cells, which serves as a transporter.

Although it has successfully captured the oxygen, hemoglobin releases the cells under particular conditions (temperature, acidity, content in carbon dioxide). If any of these conditions within tissues change, hemoglobin will not release the oxygen.

## What causes it?

Pollution, free radicals, stress, internal contamination (either snuff, alcohol, dyes and preservatives ...) age, sedentary lifestyle, chronic diseases, emotional stress, prolonged sun exposure, among others; surroundings affect the level of oxygen in our body.

### The deficit of oxygen in tissues can cause:

- A reduction in energy production.
- The biochemical reactions of assimilation and transformation of nutrients are not completed successfully.
- Waste poorly eliminated, and gradually accumulate toxicity in the body.
- The brain and the central nervous system, the largest consumers of oxygen, are the first affected. Hence alarm signals are triggered: chronic fatigue, nervousness, memory lapses... and then all body functions are affected/ diminished.

### To sum up:

Biocatalytic oxygenation helps cells assimilate oxygen more easily due to a specific and extremely reactive catalyst. This is what makes it more effective than other similar methods that can cause hyper-oxygenation, which is hardly useful, on most occasions and even damaging.

It does not have the usual inconveniences found in traditional oxygenation, and can be applied even when the latter is not advised.

IT HAS NO COUNTER-INDICATIONS, SHOWS NO TOXICITY AND IS NOT ADDICTIVE.

## ION TRANSFER

An effective pain control technique especially used for neuralgic pains. Effectiveness can be noticeable only after a few sessions and it regulates the nervous system, helps relieve respiratory diseases and induces activation of the lymphatic system's defenses. It also serves as a great support in the treatment of cardiovascular diseases, fibromyalgia and obesity, among others.

In recent years, physicists have devised many ways to use the oddities of quantum mechanics to transmit and process information.

Health is an important step to use this quantum information: transferring the quantum state of one ion to another. Since ions can store a quantum state for many seconds, this system of "quantum teleportation" could involve enough time to get the equilibrium restored in the nervous system, reduce inflammation, eliminate pain and help in the treatment of many other diseases.

The "Synmerizacion Rizada" produces a sedative and regulatory effect, including multiple pathologies derived from the nervous system. The action of the current inhibits nervous influxes exerted by the autonomic nervous system on the cerebrospinal system, regulating the neurovegetative system and, therefore, balancing the sympathetic-parasympathetic systems.

**This allows spectacular results on the following treatments:**

- Anxiety
- Migraines
- Stress
- Circulatory System
- Depression
- Dysautonomia
- Fibromyalgia
- Parkinson's Disease
- Migraines
- Multiple Sclerosis

## LIVER CLEANSE

**1) Necessary ingredients for the Liver Cleanse:** *(Total duration of treatment: 5 days)*

- THREE litres of apple juice (free from additives or artificial flavouring)
- High amounts of fruit, fresh vegetables to intake during the first 3 days (NO OTHER FOOD is allowed during the first 3 days)
- Four tablespoons of Epsom salt (MgSO4) dissolved in three glasses of water. This will be used for 4 servings, ¾ of a glass each one.
- Half a glass of Extra Virgin Olive Oil (highest quality as possible)
- Grapefruit juice*, hand-squeezed (preferrably pink but any other will do) to fill up half a glass.

*\*If you find it difficult to find grapefruit, you may use lemons even though grapefruit juice will mix much better with oil.*

**2) Preparation:**

Although not essential, it would be of great help having a colon hydrotherapy the same morning you plan on starting the liquid diet or the day before.

**Days 1, 2 & 3**

During the preparation phase of our liver cleansing, we must have a liquid diet during 3 consecutive days. Food may be steamed, raw or cooked and in any case liquefied as a shake. They may be room temperature juices or hot soups too.

If you have a portion every half an hour you would need about 20kg of fruit and vegetables per day.

It is suggested that fruit juices and shakes should be consumed only during the morning (except apple juice, which may be taken also during the evening). You may have 1L of apple juice daily during the following 3 days after 3pm, besides vegetable soups and shakes, the more quantity, the better. It is convenient not to have cold juice (best to keep them room temperature.) Do not ingest any kind of solid food. You may also have water and tea.

**Day 4**

Ideally you should have a light breakfast without butter, sugars or milk. Instead, fresh fruit and juices. Eat steamed vegetables with white rice (preferably basmati) or potatoes, i.e. avoiding proteins (you may add some Herbamare or Himalayan salt for seasoning, nothing else).

- **After 14:00h:** Do not eat or drink anything (except water) and follow the recommendations at each time of the day strictly. Until 18:00h HAVE ABSOLUTELY NOTHING.

- **18:00h:** Add three glasses of water to an empty container, dissolve 4 flat tablespoons of Epsom salts. We will divide the mixture to drink it in 4 doses (4 glasses). Now drink the 1st DOSE (you may drink water afterwards to help clear the bitter taste it may have).

- **20:00h:** 2nd DOSE of water with Epsom salts.

- **21:30h:** If you have not evacuated yet and have not done the colon hydrotherapy the preceding 24 hours, have an enema done containing warm water with a few drops of lemon (this will help to evacuate). Evacuation is necessary before proceeding with the liver cleansing.

- **21:45h:** Clean grapefruits or lemons, squeeze them manually and remove the pulp. You will need 1/2 cup of juice and 1/2 cup of oil. Mix vigorously until the mixture is apparently homogeneous. This mixture should be taken at 22:00, but if you need to go to the toilet a few times, you may delay it up to 10 minutes.

- **22:00h:** Standing up next to your bed (do not sit down), drink the mixture. Some prefer taking it with a straw. Don't take longer than 5 minutes in drinking it. Immediately after this, stretch out in bed.

**Important:** Do not move at all during the first 20 minutes in bed, as if you were a statue. Turn the lights off and place the head higher up than the belly/gut. If you are feeling uncomfortable, stretch through your right side with bent knees and your head facing towards your knees (fetal position). Stay this way for 20 minutes without talking. Fix your attention towards your liver and how clean it will be after all the hard work.

You may feel the stones moving through the bile ducts as if they were marbles. You will not feel pain due to the Magnesium in Epsom salts (keeps the bile ducts well dilated and relaxed as well has bile secretion lubricating the ducts as the stones pass by). It is recommended that you try to sleep. If you feel the urge to evacuate during the night you must do so. Check for small green/light brown pea-like stones floating in the toilet.

You may feel mild dizziness and/or nausea (occurs in 10% of cases) due to the cleanse overnight or early in the morning. This is due to the sudden heavy discharge of toxins from the liver and gallbladder that push the oil mixture down into the intestine. These feelings will dwindle throughout the morning.

## Day 5

- **Starting at 6:00h:** (or the time you prefer but not earlier than 6:00h): After waking up, drink the 3rd DOSE of Epsom Salts (if you feel thirsty, drink a glass of room temperature water before taking the dose). Relax, read, meditate, and if you feel tired, go back to bed and rest (even though it is preferable to have the body standing in a vertical position). Most people feel fine and would rather do gentle exercises.

- **8:00h:** (or 2 hours after the third dose): Drink the 4th DOSE of Epsom salts.

- **10:00h:** (or 2 hours after the fourth and last dose): You may drink fresh juice at this time. Half an hour later, you may eat one or two pieces of fresh fruit and an hour later solid food (not in big quantities).

- **In the evening or the next morning** you will begin to feel normal again and notice the first signs of improvement after this cure or liver/gallbladder cleanse. Continue with a light diet during the two following days.

**NOTES:** It would be normal to suffer diarrhea during the morning of the 5th day. You may find stones in the toilet after evacuating. The interesting ones are green in color since this indicates they are gallstones. These stones will usually float due to their high content in cholesterol. It would be a good idea to count them all (whether green or not). The optimum point is reached when there is a total of 2000+/- stones, enough to relieve the organism from discomfort, back aches and/or allergies, bursitis and headaches. Never do this cleanse when being sick, and in all cases, we recommend checking with your doctor, therapist or any other qualified health professional. The information contained in this section is for informative purposes only.

## LOW FREQUENCY LASER

The low-power laser provides a refreshing and beneficial effect on the nervous tissue, skeletal muscle, soft tissue and skin.

From the biochemical point of view, its main action lies in the modulation of oxidative phosphorylation at the mitochondrial level, where the synthesis of adenosine triphosphate (ATP) is stimulated, which is the fundamental form of energy of the cell.

This therapy is indicated for any systemic disease, febrile inflammation, pain, and tissue repair disorders.

The duration of the treatment depends on the doctor's decision you will not feel any discomfort, and it doesn't have secondary effects.

## OZONE THERAPY

Ozone acts as an antioxidant and immunomodulator (stimulates white blood cells, which increases the body's defenses against external agents such as infections and as a detector of mutagenic cells which cause cancer or autoimmune diseases). In addition, the level of red blood cells that release oxygen increases, leading to greater oxygen transport to the cells, therefore improving cellular function and overall circulation.

It is also a powerful germicide: eliminates fungi, bacteria and viruses.

These set of benefits make therapeutic applications have a wide range of treatments, treating various diseases (from carcinomas; cerebral sclerosis and Parkinson's; to cystitis, circulatory disorders, liver cirrhosis, hepatitis and gallbladder diseases).

Rheumatic diseases in general, polyarthrosis, herniated discs, arthritis, thrombophlebitis and varicose veins are also covered. Gangrene and diabetic ulcers; ulcerative colitis, irritable colon, anal eczema, anal fissures and fistulas, hemorrhoids and genital infections.

Ozone improves our metabolism noticeably. On the one hand, it improves blood circulation in the affected tissues, and on the other hand, the transport of oxygen and, therefore, the power supply to swollen or affected areas is improved. The immune system is positively stimulated. On top of these effects, in the field of cosmetics, ozone acts as a powerful skin cell activator and is also used as a potent immunostimulating, anti-inflammatory and pain deactivator.

**In conclusion:**
- It activates the immune system in infectious diseases.
- It improves the cellular utilization of oxygen that reduces ischemia in cardiovascular diseases, and in many of the infirmities of aging.
- It causes the release of growth factors that stimulate damaged joints and degenerative discs to regenerate.
- It can dramatically reduce or even eliminate many cases of chronic pain through its action on pain receptors.
- Published papers have demonstrated its healing effects on interstitial cystitis, chronic hepatitis, herpes infections, dental infections, diabetes, and macular degeneration.

## PAPIMI ELECTROMAGNETIC IMPULSES

*Papimi is a high end device that is inducing electromagnetic impulses directly into the somatic cell. In addition to activating the process of self-healing, papimi provides extraordinarily fast results in a wide range of applications.*

Is a non-invasive electromagnetic device that produces a series of magnetic pulses of strong but extremely short broadband.

A pulsed electromagnetic field emanating flexible papimi conductive hoop, which is placed in the body areas to be treated. The energy field penetrates deep into the tissues to relieve pain, increase circulation and help the body heal itself by energizing cells.

The injured body cells re-energize, pain signals carried by the nervous system decrease, swelling decreases, and the range of motion is restored. The toxins are released and essential nutrients for the repairing process are absorbed.

## How does it work?

The device uses a magnetic field to penetrate the body, passing right through the skin into the affected tissue(s). The magnetic field is there only for a short time but in great intensity. A magnetic field induced as papimi is able to penetrate most substances.

As the field changes during the pulses brief timelapse, expanding and collapsing in less than one ten-millionth of a second, it causes a small current that provides bioenergy to the cells in an immediate way.

The penetration depth of the induction amounts to about 20 centimeters at full power.

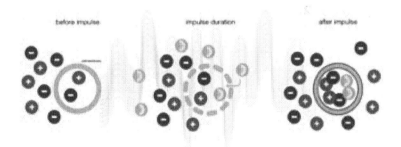

**The biological treatment of cancer with papimi pursues the following targets:**
- Reinforcement of cells and immune system
- Improvement of therapy results
- Decrease of side effects of conventional cancer therapies
- Increase of quality of life
- Stimulation of self-healing effects

## HYPERTHERMIA

### Local Deep Hyperthermia
It consists in raising the temperature of the tumor up to a maximum of 41 degrees C to 43.5 degrees C, and this damages the nucleus of the cancer cells.

Deep Local Hyperthermia is an essential tool for the treatment of cancer in conjunction with other cancer treatments (chemo and radiation) or independent of them.

### Whole Body Hyperthermia
Using infared lamps, the body temperature activating the immune system is raised (between 38 degrees C – 40 degrees C), causing an "artificial" fever.

Whole Body Hyperthermia can be used for other diseases that require an immune system activation.

## DETOX FOOT BATH

Using controlled low-voltage bio-electricity, a detox foot bath pulls toxins out of the body through the feet.

Used in conjunction with other protocols, a detox foot bath is a valuable part of overall treatment.

One of the most popular brands of detox foot bath is the *Mary Staggs Detox System.*

▶

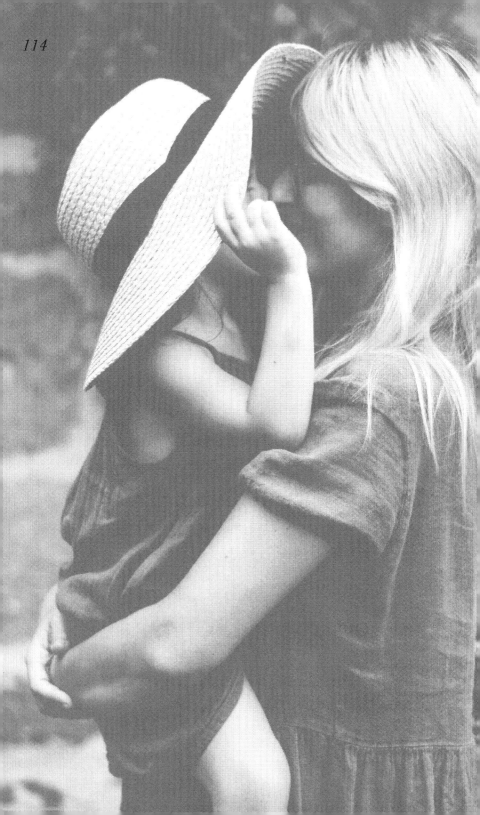

## Bonus:

# Resources
# And
# Helps ▶

*" For by wise counsel you will wage your own war, And in a multitude of counselors there is safety."*

*Proverbs 24:6*

## Having the right tools can make all the difference.

In my ongoing journey of overcoming cancer, I've spent countless hours researching, testing and using all sorts of helpful information, books, websites, medical personnel, cooking aids, supplements and more.

This is a list of some of the key resources that I continue to reference and use. Please note: There's no one perfect diet, tool or resource that is always best for everyone. However, these are things that I, and those I get to walk on this journey with, have found to be incredibly helpful.

### Food and Cooking

- *Against All Grain* by Danielle Walker
- *Cook 2 Flourish* by Robin and Julie Cook
- *Eat Dirt* by Dr. Josh Axe

### Informational Books and Websites

- *Keto Diet* by Dr. Josh Axe

- *The Ketogenic Diet* by Kristen Mancinelli
- *The Hormone Reset Diet* by Sarah Gotfried
- *The Cancer Killers* by Dr. Charles Major
- *Healthy and Free* by Beni Johnson
- *I Am Resilient* by Andrea Thompson
- Living Nutrition Plans www.maxliving.com
- www.greenmedinfo.com
- Dr. Joshua Axe www.draxe.com

**Companies and People**
- www.clinicahilu.com
- MaxLiving www.maxliving.com
- Dr. Sonja O'Bryan (email: drsonjaobryan@gmail.com)
- Dr. Bobby Fano www.verticalchiroredding.com
- 100percentpure.com
- Ashley Nelson Studios, facebook.com
- Johanna Budwig www.budwigcenter.com
- Dr. Inga Wetzel www.healthstudio.com
- Dr. Amanda Campbell, New Life Chiropractic, Lee's Summit, Missouri, 816-347-1515
- Kitchen Craft Cookware, West Bend, WI (Stainless

Steel, Waterless cookware)
- *Lodge* brand cast iron cookware (Made in USA)
- www.safesleevecases.com (smartphone cases)
- www.giawellness.com

**Supplements To Purchase**
- Nature's Sunshine Supplements: www.healthbyGod.mynsp.com
- Max Living Supplements http://store.maxliving.com/?srrf=wSAKX

▶

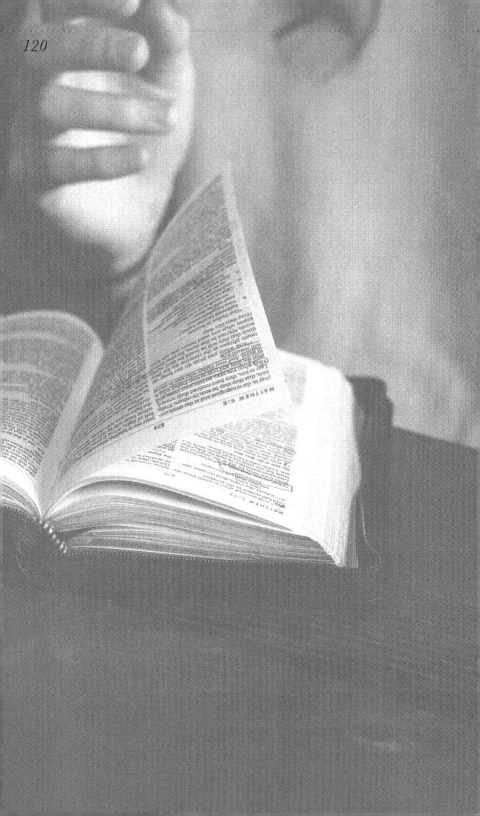

**Next Steps:**

# Where
# to Go
# From Here ▶

*"If you need wisdom, ask our generous God, and he will give it to you. He will not rebuke you for asking."*

*James 1:5*

## Cancer is a harsh reality to be faced with.

The painful reality is that cancer affects men, women and children. According to the American Cancer Society, in 2019, there will be an estimated 1,762,450 new cancer cases diagnosed and 606,880 cancer deaths in the United States. This means that over 1600 people will die today because of cancer!

I was talking with a friend and I was describing what it was like walking through cancer. I felt like when I received my diagnosis, I had become dead. My spirit, soul and body felt close to death, and through the power of God, He allowed me to watch Him resurrect me back to life. Even though the journey was hard, it was the greatest honor to be able to partner with God and watch Him bring me back to life before I even reached the grave! That's the power of God at work!

My journey is far from over. You see, I realized that we are all fighting for our lives every day. As I mentioned in the opening chapter, I didn't just get cancer one day. It had been living inside of me for over ten years! My body is now cancer-free, but that doesn't give me the free pass to stop living from a place of victory!

> *My body is now cancer-free, but that doesn't give me the free pass to stop living from a place of victory!*

I learned that there is a vast difference between fighting for your health from a place of rest and fighting from a place of chaos. When I had cancer, I was fighting from a place of chaos because my life was on the line. Now I still fight every single day, but from a place of rest.

We are living in a world full of toxins and foods that are making us sick. Everyday, something tries to come at us to jeopardize our health and wellness. I would rather be preventative and on guard to these things instead of choosing to look the other way hoping that nothing happens.

I've learned that maintaining our health is similar to maintaining our relationship with God. We shouldn't just read the Bible when we are in an emergency. We should be reading every day to fill our spirits with hope and life. That way when the enemy comes to kill, steal, and destroy, we are already prepared with weapons in our arsenal. We need to have this same mindset when it comes to our health. We need to be choosing life every day for our bodies.

I want to encourage you reading this that my journey was a process. I never expected to be diagnosed with cancer, so I was in uncharted waters when it came to recovery. I was thrown into a world that I never wanted to be a part of. It's easy to fall into the victim mindset and get to the place where you want to just throw your hands in the air and yell, "I guess this cancer is my destiny!"

## Cancer is not your destiny!

Yes, it's scary and overwhelming to the point where you can feel hopeless, but you were created to be an overcomer! If you or a loved one is struggling with cancer, know that I was just like you. I was faced with a paralyzing fear that I had to choose to overcome.

I learned in my journey that it was okay to seek out help and to allow the Lord to lead me to people who could help me. I gave myself over to the process and fully trusted those God had placed in my life to help me overcome.

My next piece of advice is to not stop taking care of your body just because you feel better! It's important to not recreate the environment that created cancer in the first place. I know that this may sound like common sense, but the truth is that I see it happen all the time. People ask me, "How long do I have to do this for?" My response always is, "Every day that you want to be healthy." Keep in mind that it's been proven that 98% of all disease is due to lifestyle![1]

If we want to overcome cancer and sustain our breakthrough, we have to make these changes a lifestyle. My favorite saying I learned from my health coach Robin Cook is "alteration, not deprivation." We cannot live our lives afraid to enjoy food again; we just have to learn new habits. During my journey, my daughter began experimenting in the kitchen and created recipes that could be enjoyed and savored while still honoring our health. There are many beautiful cookbooks that you can utilize to help inspire you and keep you healthy at the same time.

My journey in overcoming cancer demonstrated to me, and now to thousands of others, that defeating

---

1        http://drleaf.com/blog/you-are-what-you-think-75-98-of-mental-and-physical-illnesses-come-from-our-thought-life/

cancer really was possible. As you can see in the pages that you just read in this book, there was a pathway for me to overcome.

Don't settle for cancer having to be a death sentence for you or for someone you know and love. My prayer is that you have experienced hope for your journey in the short time we've been together.

It's an absolute privilege and honor to be able to encourage you in this process.

*I'd love to connect with you:*

andreathompson.org

info@andreathompson.org

## Other books by Andrea Thompson

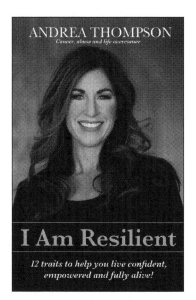

In *I Am Resilient*, cancer, abuse and life overcomer Andrea Thompson gives a refreshing perspective to the idea of resilience, and how it's not about just trying harder. Through her own experiences, involving both failure and success, Andrea unveils 12 keys that are a part of a person's persona who wants to overcome any type of setback or challenge, and build a successful journey that defies the odds and brings lasting happiness, hope and real-life results.

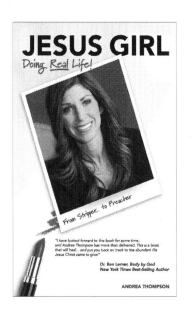

*Jesus Girl - Doing Real Life* tells the heartfelt story of one woman's journey from a lost life as a stripper...through her struggles with abusive relationships...to her salvation and redemption with the help and support of a strong and loving Christian community. Proving that anything is possible when one's life is guided by Jesus Christ, Andrea Thompson lays out direct and insightful advice on how each of us can help those around us find a better way with God's Good Guidance.